I0765930

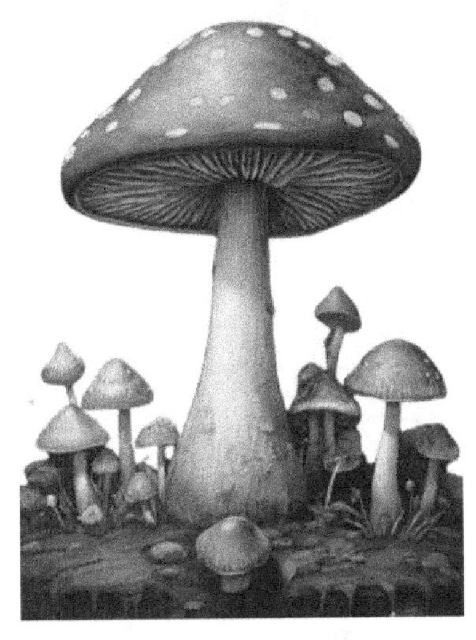

THE ULTIMATE GUIDE TO DIY MUSHROOM CHOCOLATE AND COFFEE ELIXIRS

UNLOCKING NATURE'S BREW – TRANSFORM YOUR DAILY RITUALS WITH FLAVORFUL ALCHEMY AND WELLNESS WONDERS

A J BLAZE

DISCLAIMER

The information provided in this book, "THE ULTIMATE GUIDE TO DIY MUSHROOM CHOCOLATE AND COFFEE ELIXIRS," is intended for educational and informational purposes only. The content of this book is not intended to be a substitute for professional medical advice, diagnosis, or treatment. The usage and consumption of mushroom chocolate and coffee elixirs involve inherent risks, and it is important to consult with a qualified healthcare professional before embarking on any new dietary or wellness regimen.

The author and publisher of this book are not responsible for any adverse effects, consequences, or damages resulting from the use or misuse of the information provided. The reader must assume full responsibility for their own actions, choices, and decisions based on the information presented in this book.

Furthermore, the recipes, techniques, and suggestions discussed in this book may require special equipment or ingredients that could pose risks if improperly handled or used. It is essential to follow all safety precautions, manufacturer instructions, and local regulations while preparing and consuming these mushroom chocolate and coffee elixirs.

Individual experiences may vary, and the effectiveness of these elixirs may differ for each person. Readers are encouraged to conduct their own research, exercise caution, and consult professionals when necessary.

By purchasing and reading this book,you acknowledge that you have read, understood, and agreed to the terms and disclaimers stated above. You agree to hold the author and publisher harmless from any claims, damages, or injuries that may arise as a result of the use of the information provided in this book.

Contents

INTRODUCTION

Welcome to the World of Mushroom-Infused Indulgences—a realm where culinary creativity intertwines with holistic wellness. This introduction sets the stage for an enlightening journey into the fusion of mushrooms, chocolate, and coffee, inviting readers to explore the captivating synergy between these elements.

Within these pages lies a treasure trove of knowledge and inspiration, curated to tantalize taste buds, nourish curiosity, and delve into the health-conscious realm of homemade delights. Here, we embark on a voyage that transcends traditional culinary boundaries, embracing the earthy, aromatic world of mushrooms as they intertwine harmoniously with the decadence of chocolate and the boldness of coffee.

This introduction aims to bridge the gap between the familiar and the unexplored, inviting both novices and aficionados into this innovative culinary landscape. It elucidates the transformative potential of mushrooms, transcending their conventional roles as savory ingredients to become exquisite companions to the realm of indulgent treats.

We'll unravel the secrets behind selecting the finest mushrooms, uncover the artistry of infusing their essence into chocolate and coffee elixirs, and unlock the myriad health benefits these mushrooms offer. Together, we'll discover how these homemade infusions can elevate not just taste, but overall well-being.

Prepare to be enchanted by the nuanced flavors, nourished by their potential health benefits, and empowered to craft your own delectable creations. Join us on this voyage as we navigate the tantalizing world of Mushroom-Infused Indulgences, where creativity meets wellness, and the familiar meets the extraordinary. Let's embark on a journey that celebrates innovation, fosters curiosity, and elevates the everyday—welcome to a world where mushrooms, chocolate, and coffee converge in exquisite harmony.

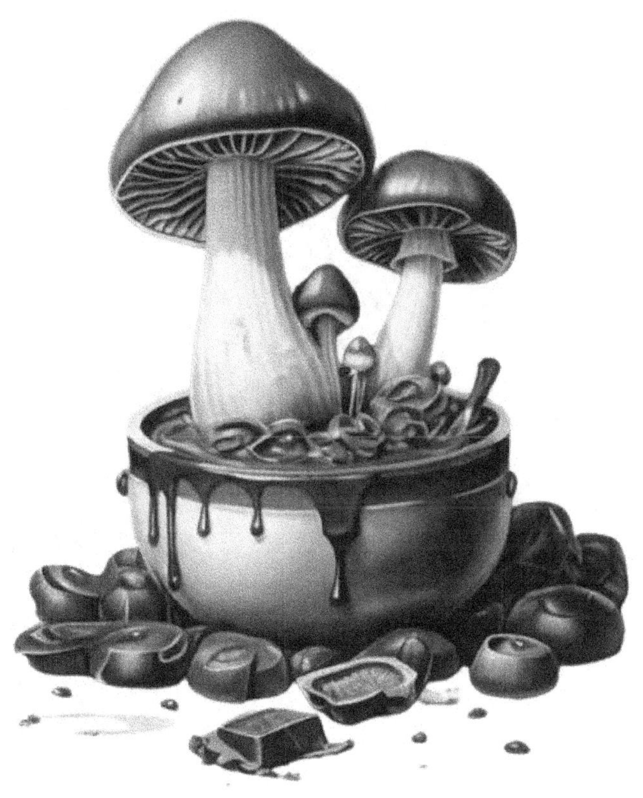

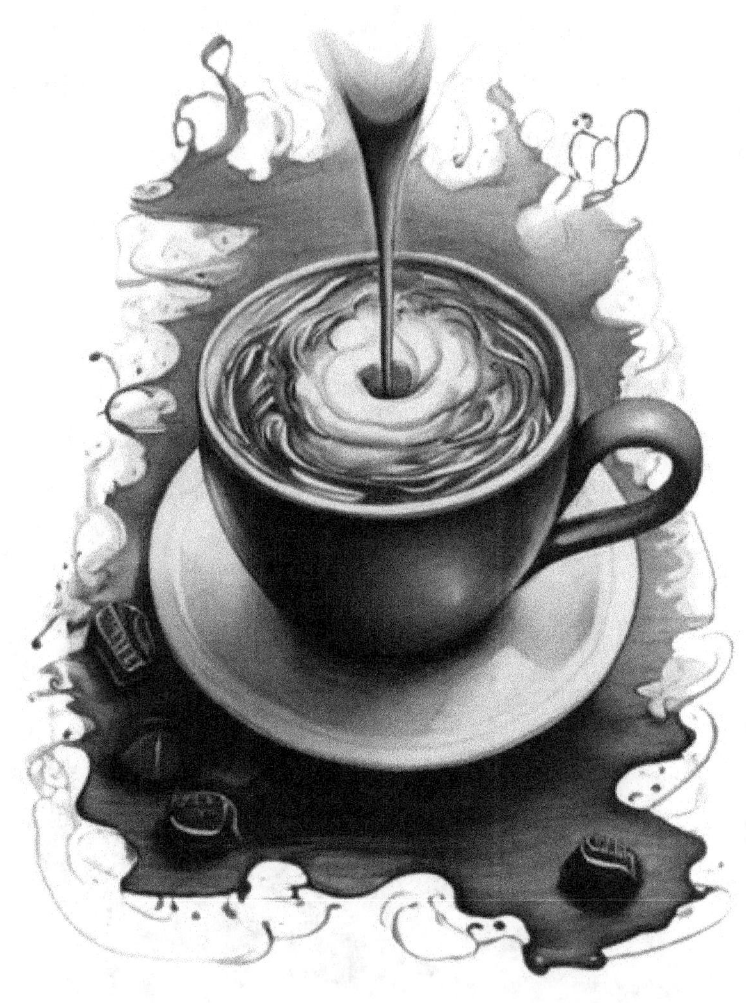

UNDERSTANDING THE HEALTH BENEFITS AND CULINARY POTENTIAL OF MUSHROOMS

Understanding the health benefits and culinary potential of mushrooms unveils a world of nutritional richness and gastronomic versatility. Beyond their earthy flavors and varied textures, mushrooms harbor a treasure trove of wellness-enhancing properties that elevate them from mere ingredients to nutritional powerhouses.

NUTRITIONAL PROFICIENCY OF MUSHROOMS

Mushrooms are a source of essential nutrients, including vitamins, minerals, and antioxidants. They offer an array of B vitamins, notably riboflavin (B2), niacin (B3), and pantothenic acid (B5), vital for energy production and overall well-being. Their mineral content includes selenium, copper, potassium, and phosphorus, contributing to immune support, cell function, and bone health.

Medicinal Potency and Health Benefits

Numerous mushroom species boast medicinal properties that have fascinated cultures worldwide for centuries. Varieties like reishi, lion's mane, and chaga exhibit immune-boosting, anti-inflammatory, and adaptogenic qualities. They are revered for their potential to support mental clarity, stress reduction, and even cardiovascular health.

Culinary Versatility and Flavor Enhancement

Mushrooms offer a canvas for culinary innovation, adding depth, umami richness, and distinctive flavors to dishes. Their versatility allows for diverse cooking methods—whether sautéed, grilled, roasted, or incorporated raw into salads. From the meaty texture of portobellos to the delicate nature of enoki mushrooms, each variety offers a unique taste profile, enhancing a wide range of dishes.

Mushroom Infusions: A Fusion of Taste and Wellness

Infusing mushrooms into chocolate and coffee amplifies both taste and health benefits. The inherent earthiness of mushrooms complements the sweetness of chocolate and the robustness of coffee, creating an indulgent yet health-conscious fusion. This unique combination offers an innovative approach to incorporating mushrooms into daily consumption, appealing to both culinary enthusiasts and wellness-conscious individuals.

Understanding the holistic potential of mushrooms—nourishing the body, tantalizing the palate, and supporting overall well-being—paves the way for an enlightening exploration into the realms of Mushroom-Infused Indulgences. It sets the foundation for embracing their multifaceted role in culinary creativity, wellness, and the fusion of flavor and nutrition.

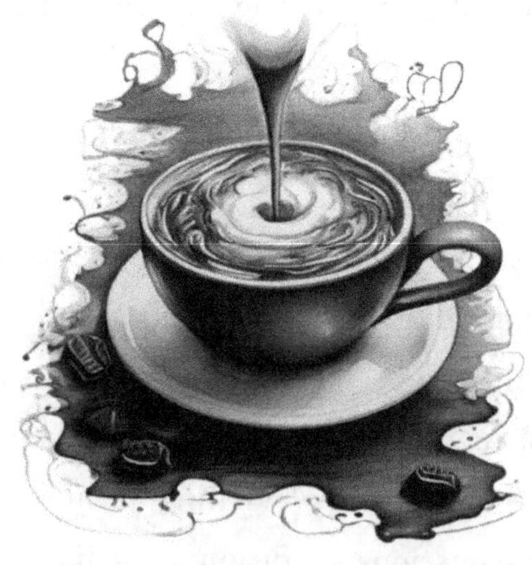

CHAPTER 1: EXPLORING MUSHROOM VARIETIES

1.1 An Overview of Medicinal Mushrooms for Culinary Use

An overview of medicinal mushrooms for culinary use reveals a diverse spectrum of fungi with profound health benefits and versatile culinary applications. These mushrooms, renowned for their therapeutic properties, offer a captivating blend of flavor, nutrition, and potential wellness support when incorporated into culinary creations.

REISHI (GANODERMA LUCIDUM)

Reishi stands as a revered mushroom in traditional Chinese medicine, celebrated for its adaptogenic qualities. Its bitter profile blends well with savory dishes and infusions, offering immune-boosting and stress-reducing properties.

LION'S MANE (HERICIUM ERINACEUS)

Known for its unique appearance resembling a lion's mane, this mushroom exhibit potential cognitive benefits, supporting brain health and nerve regeneration. Its delicate, seafood-like flavor suits both savory dishes and sweet infusions.

CHAGA (INONOTUS OBLIQUUS)

Chaga, with its dark, woody exterior, contains antioxidants and immune-enhancing compounds. Its earthy, slightly bitter taste complements coffee or chocolate infusions, lending depth and health benefits.

CORDYCEPS (CORDYCEPS MILITARIS)

Cordyceps mushrooms, historically used in traditional medicine, offer potential energy-boosting properties and endurance support. Their mild, nutty flavor suits various culinary creations, from soups to beverages.

TURKEY TAIL (TRAMETES VERSICOLOR)

Named for its colorful bands resembling a turkey's tail, this mushroom is rich in polysaccharides with immune-supportive attributes. Its subtle flavor makes it adaptable for infusions or as a culinary complement.

SHIITAKE (LENTINULA EDODES)

A culinary favorite, shiitake mushrooms boast immune-boosting properties and a robust, meaty flavor. Widely used in savory dishes, their versatility extends to enhancing chocolate-based recipes.

MAITAKE (GRIFOLA FRONDOSA)

Maitake mushrooms offer immune-modulating potential and a unique texture reminiscent of hen-of-the-woods. Their earthy, umami-rich taste pairs well with chocolate infusions or savory dishes.

PORCINI (BOLETUS EDULIS)

Porcini mushrooms, esteemed for their robust, nutty flavor, enrich dishes with antioxidants and potential anti-inflammatory properties. Their earthy taste complements both sweet and savory infusions.

Exploring the culinary potential and medicinal attributes of these mushrooms invites a holistic understanding of their multifaceted nature. Integrating these fungi into culinary creations not only offers unique flavors but also introduces a spectrum of potential health benefits, fostering a harmonious fusion of taste and well-being.

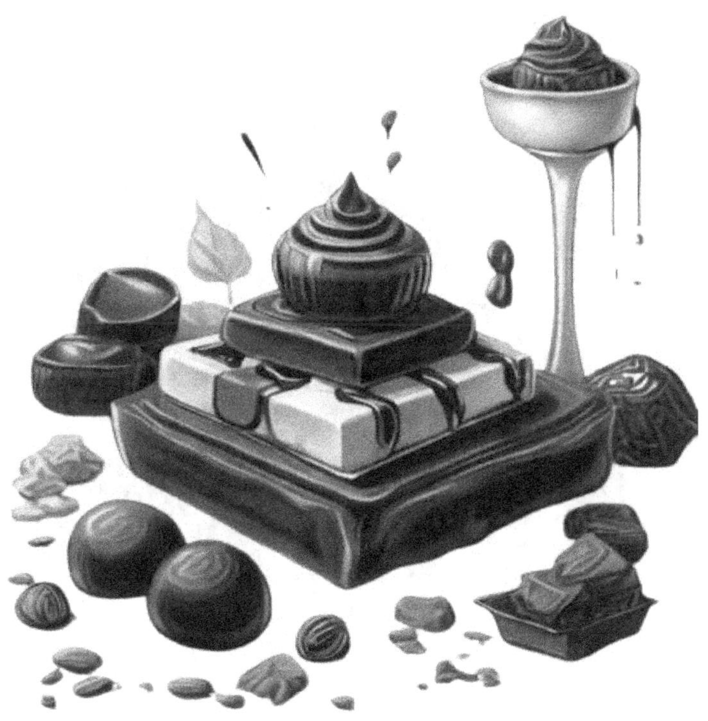

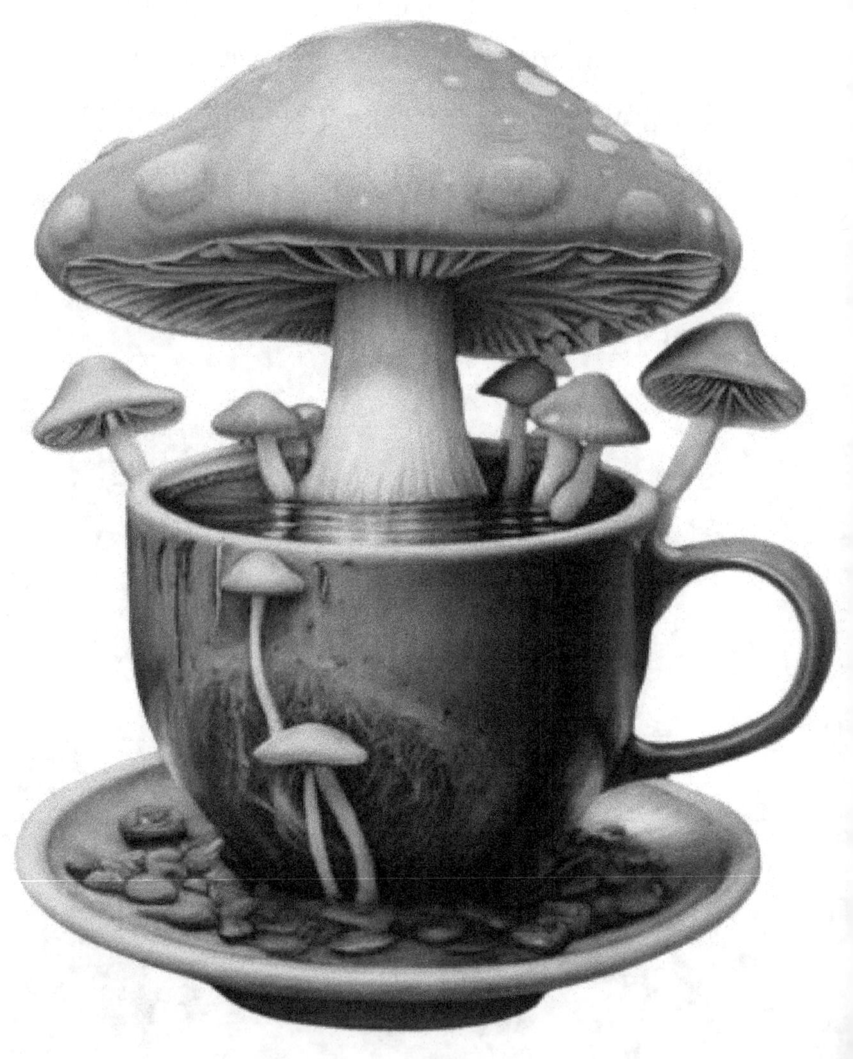

1.2 Selecting the Right Mushrooms for Chocolate and Coffee Infusions

Selecting the right mushrooms for chocolate and coffee infusions involves a nuanced understanding of mushroom varieties, flavor profiles, and their compatibility with these indulgent treats. This selection process not only enhances taste but also amplifies potential health benefits, offering a harmonious blend of culinary delight and wellness support.

UNDERSTANDING FLAVOR PROFILES

Each mushroom boasts distinct flavor characteristics, ranging from earthy and nutty to bitter or subtly sweet. For chocolate and coffee infusions, consider mushrooms that complement the flavors without overpowering the inherent taste of the treats.

COMPLEMENTING TASTE AND AROMA

Opt for mushrooms that harmonize with the inherent flavors of chocolate and coffee. Mushrooms like reishi, with its mild bitterness, pair well with the rich sweetness of chocolate, while the subtle, earthy notes of lion's mane or chaga can enhance the robustness of coffee without overshadowing its aroma.

CONSIDERING CULINARY VERSATILITY

Versatile mushrooms like shiitake, maitake, or porcini offer adaptability in culinary applications, seamlessly integrating into chocolate-based recipes or enriching coffee infusions with their unique flavors. Their compatibility with various culinary creations makes them suitable candidates for experimentation.

PRIORITIZING MEDICINAL ATTRIBUTES

Mushrooms renowned for their medicinal properties, such as reishi or chaga, bring an additional layer of health benefits to the infusion process. Their potential immune-boosting, stress-reducing, or antioxidant-rich properties elevate the overall wellness quotient of the chocolate and coffee blends.

SUITABILITY FOR INFUSION METHODS

Consider the suitability of mushrooms for infusion techniques. Some mushrooms, like lion's mane or cordyceps, lend themselves well to extraction methods, allowing their beneficial compounds to infuse seamlessly into chocolate or coffee.

QUALITY AND SOURCING

Emphasize sourcing high-quality mushrooms from reputable sources to ensure purity and potency. Fresh, dried, or powdered forms of mushrooms can be selected based on availability and intended infusion techniques.

Selecting the right mushrooms for chocolate and coffee infusions involves a delicate balance between flavor, culinary adaptability, and potential health attributes. By carefully considering these factors, enthusiasts can craft enticing and health-conscious creations that elevate the taste and nutritional value of these beloved treats.

MUSHROOMS FOR CHOCOLATE INFUSIONS:

REISHI (GANODERMA LUCIDUM):

Flavor Profile: Mild bitterness with subtle earthy undertones.

Chocolate Pairing: Complements the sweetness of chocolate while adding depth to its flavor.

Benefits: Immune-boosting properties and stress-reducing potential.

LION'S MANE (HERICIUM ERINACEUS):

Flavor Profile: Delicate and slightly sweet, reminiscent of seafood.

Chocolate Pairing: Blends well with the richness of chocolate, offering a unique flavor profile.

Benefits: Potential cognitive support and nerve-regenerative properties.

CHAGA (INONOTUS OBLIQUUS):

Flavor Profile: Earthy and slightly bitter.

Chocolate Pairing: Enhances the depth of chocolate flavor without overpowering sweetness.

Benefits: Antioxidant-rich and immune-enhancing qualities.

MUSHROOMS FOR COFFEE INFUSIONS:

LION'S MANE (HERICIUM ERINACEUS):

Flavor Profile: Delicate and slightly sweet, akin to seafood.

Coffee Pairing: Blends well with coffee's robustness, adding a subtle earthiness.

Benefits: Potential cognitive support and adaptogenic properties.

CORDYCEPS (CORDYCEPS MILITARIS):

Flavor Profile: Mild, nutty taste.

Coffee Pairing: Harmonizes with coffee's flavor, potentially boosting energy and endurance.

Benefits: Potential energy-boosting properties and endurance support.

CHAGA (INONOTUS OBLIQUUS):

Flavor Profile: Earthy and slightly bitter.
Coffee Pairing: Complements coffee's boldness, adding depth and richness.

Benefits: Antioxidant-rich and potential immune-enhancing properties.

These mushrooms exhibit diverse flavors and potential health benefits that can enhance both chocolate and coffee infusions. Whether selecting mushrooms for their flavor profiles or their wellness attributes, these varieties offer a versatile range of options for crafting delightful and health-conscious infusions.

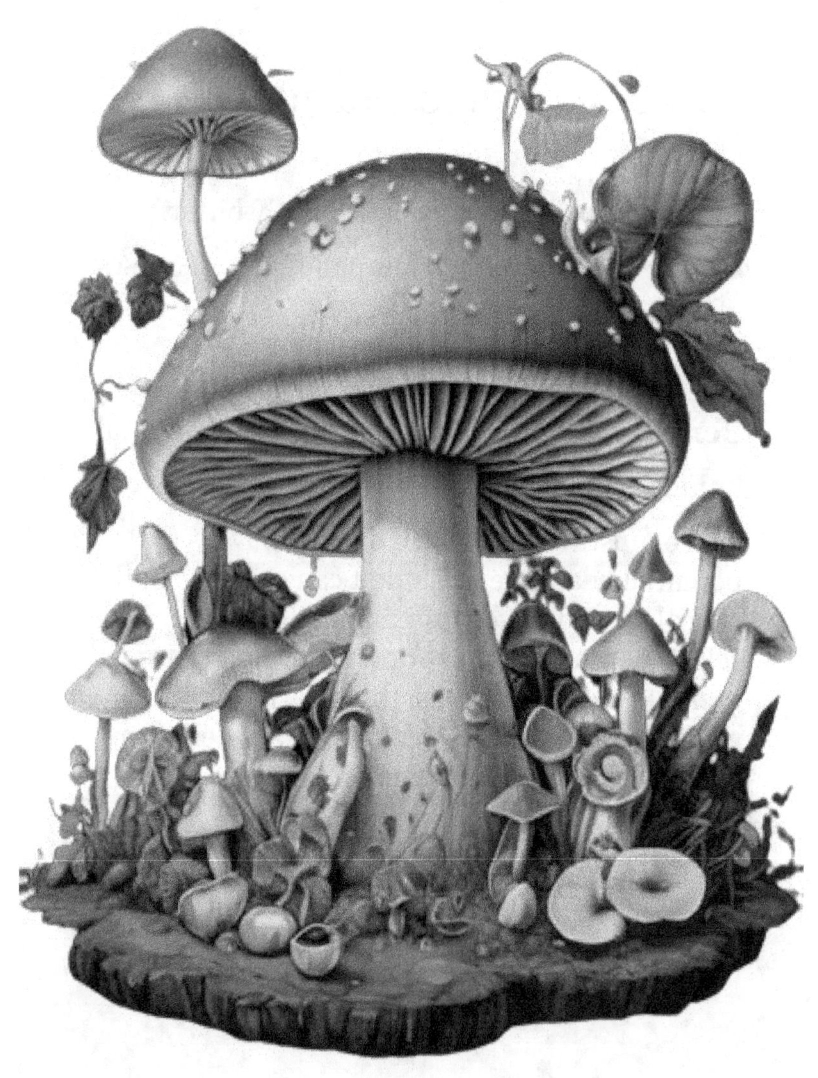

Chapter 2: The Art of Mushroom Chocolate

2.1 Basics of Homemade Chocolate Making

INGREDIENTS AND EQUIPMENT:

Cacao Beans: The foundation of chocolate, sourced from cacao pods. They can be raw or roasted, offering distinct flavor profiles.

Sweeteners: Sugar, honey, agave, or alternative sweeteners to balance the bitterness of cacao.

Cocoa Butter: The fat extracted from cacao beans, contributes to the texture and smoothness of chocolate.

Flavor Enhancers: Vanilla, sea salt, spices, or nuts for added flavor depth.

Grinder/Melanger: Essential equipment to grind and refine cacao beans into a smooth paste.

Tempering Tools: Crucial for achieving the right texture and shine in finished chocolate, including a thermometer and molds.

CHOCOLATE MAKING PROCESS:

Roasting and Grinding: Roast cacao beans to develop flavors, then crack and winnow them to separate the nibs from the shells. Grind nibs into a paste using a melanger until smooth.

Refining and Conching: Continuously grind the paste to refine particle size and release cocoa butter, leading to smoother texture. Conching involves aerating and smoothing the mixture for hours or days for optimal flavor development.

Tempering: Heat and cool chocolate to specific temperatures, aligning the cocoa butter crystals for a glossy finish and snap. This process is crucial for achieving the desired texture and avoiding a dull appearance or grainy texture.

Molding and Setting: Pour the tempered chocolate into molds, tapping to remove air bubbles. Allow it to set at controlled temperatures for the ideal texture.

TIPS FOR HOMEMADE CHOCOLATE:

Quality Ingredients: Use high-quality cacao beans and cocoa butter for superior flavor.

Temperature Control: Precision in tempering and controlled melting temperatures is key for the perfect texture.

Patience and Practice: Chocolate making is an art; refining techniques with each batch enhances the quality of the final product.

Mastering the basics of homemade chocolate-making empowers enthusiasts to craft artisanal chocolates with unique flavors, textures, and a personal touch. It's a rewarding journey that blends science, artistry, and culinary finesse.

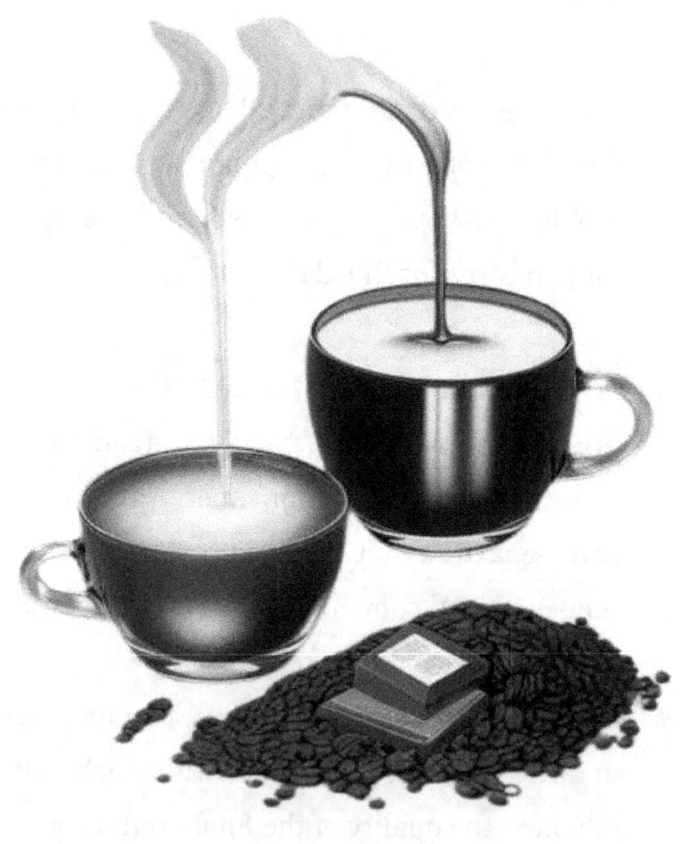

2.2 Infusing Mushroom Extracts into Chocolate Blends

HERE'S A STEP-BY-STEP GUIDE ON INFUSING MUSHROOM EXTRACTS INTO CHOCOLATE BLENDS:

MATERIALS NEEDED:

Mushroom Extract: Prepared mushroom extract of your choice (reishi, lion's mane, chaga, etc.).

Tempered Chocolate: High-quality tempered chocolate suitable for melting and molding.

Double Boiler or Microwave: For melting chocolate gently.

Mold: Chocolate molds for shaping the infused chocolate.

STEP-BY-STEP PROCESS:

1. Prepare Your Mushroom Extract:

Ensure you have your preferred mushroom extract ready for infusion.

This extract can be homemade or store-bought, prepared according to recommended instructions.

2. Melt the Chocolate:

Using a double boiler or microwave, gently melt the tempered chocolate. Stir occasionally to ensure even melting and avoid overheating.

3. Incorporate Mushroom Extract:

Once the chocolate is completely melted, add the desired amount of mushroom extract to the melted chocolate. Start with a small quantity and adjust to taste preference and potency.

Stir the mixture thoroughly to ensure the mushroom extract is evenly distributed throughout the chocolate.

4. Temper the Chocolate (if necessary):

If the addition of the mushroom extract affects the chocolate's temperature, you might need to temper it again to achieve the desired texture and shine. Follow tempering guidelines for the specific type of chocolate used.

5. Pour into Molds:

Carefully pour the infused chocolate mixture into the molds. Tap the molds gently on a flat surface to release any air bubbles and ensure even distribution.

6. Allow to Set:

Place the filled molds in a cool, dry place or the refrigerator for the chocolate to set completely. Follow the recommended temperature and timing for the proper setting.

7. Unmold and Enjoy:

Once the chocolate has solidified and set, remove the molded chocolates from the molds. Handle them carefully to prevent breakage.

Your mushroom-infused chocolate treats are now ready to be savored!

TIPS:

Experiment with different mushroom extracts and chocolate ratios to find the desired flavor and potency.

Be mindful of the mushroom extract's concentration to avoid overpowering the chocolate's taste.

Store the infused chocolates in a cool, dry place to maintain their quality.

Infusing mushroom extracts into chocolate blends offers a unique way to combine the health benefits of mushrooms with the indulgence of chocolate, creating delightful treats with added wellness attributes.

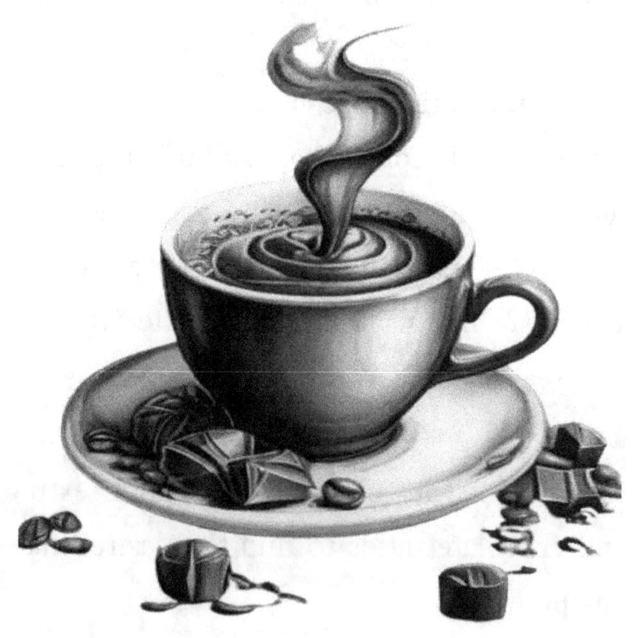

HERE ARE RECIPES FOR MUSHROOM-INFUSED CHOCOLATE BARS, TRUFFLES, AND DESSERTS:

MUSHROOM-INFUSED CHOCOLATE BARS:

INGREDIENTS:

200g high-quality dark chocolate (70% cocoa or higher)

1 tablespoon of mushroom extract (choose your preferred variety)

Optional: Nuts, dried fruits, or sea salt for additional flavor (if desired)

Instructions:

Prepare the Chocolate:

Melt the dark chocolate using a double boiler or microwave, ensuring it's smooth and fully melted.

Incorporate Mushroom Extract:

Once melted, stir in the mushroom extract thoroughly until well combined.

Add Optional Ingredients (if desired):

If using nuts, dried fruits, or sea salt, mix them into the chocolate mixture evenly.

Pour into Mold:

Pour the infused chocolate mixture into molds, spreading it evenly. Tap the molds gently to remove air bubbles.

Set and Chill:

Allow the chocolate to set in the refrigerator for about 1-2 hours until completely solidified.

Unmold and Enjoy:

Once set, remove the chocolate bars from the molds and store them in a cool, dry place.

MUSHROOM-INFUSED CHOCOLATE TRUFFLES:

INGREDIENTS:

250g dark chocolate (70% cocoa or higher), finely chopped

1/2 cup heavy cream

2 tablespoons of mushroom extract

Cocoa powder, shredded coconut, or chopped nuts for coating.

INSTRUCTIONS:

Prepare Ganache:

Heat the heavy cream until it simmers, then pour it over the finely chopped chocolate in a bowl. Let it sit for a minute, then stir until smooth.

Add Mushroom Extract:

Stir in the mushroom extract thoroughly into the ganache mixture.

Chill the Ganache:

Cover the ganache and refrigerate until firm, typically for 2-3 hours or overnight.

Form Truffles:

Scoop a spoonful of the chilled ganache and roll them into small balls. Roll the truffles in cocoa powder, shredded coconut, or chopped nuts for coating.

Chill and Serve:

Place the coated truffles on a baking sheet and refrigerate for 30 minutes before serving. Store any leftovers in the refrigerator.

MUSHROOM-INFUSED CHOCOLATE DESSERT (CHOCOLATE MOUSSE):

INGREDIENTS:

150g dark chocolate, melted

1 cup heavy cream

2 tablespoons mushroom extract

Optional: Berries or whipped cream for garnish

INSTRUCTIONS:

Prepare Chocolate Base:

Melt the dark chocolate and set it aside to cool slightly.

Whip the Cream:

Whip the heavy cream until stiff peaks form.

Combine Chocolate and Cream:

Gently fold the melted chocolate and mushroom extract into the whipped cream until well incorporated.

Chill and Serve:

Divide the chocolate mousse into serving bowls or glasses. Refrigerate for at least 2 hours before serving.

Garnish with berries or whipped cream before serving if desired.

These recipes offer delightful ways to incorporate mushroom extracts into chocolate,

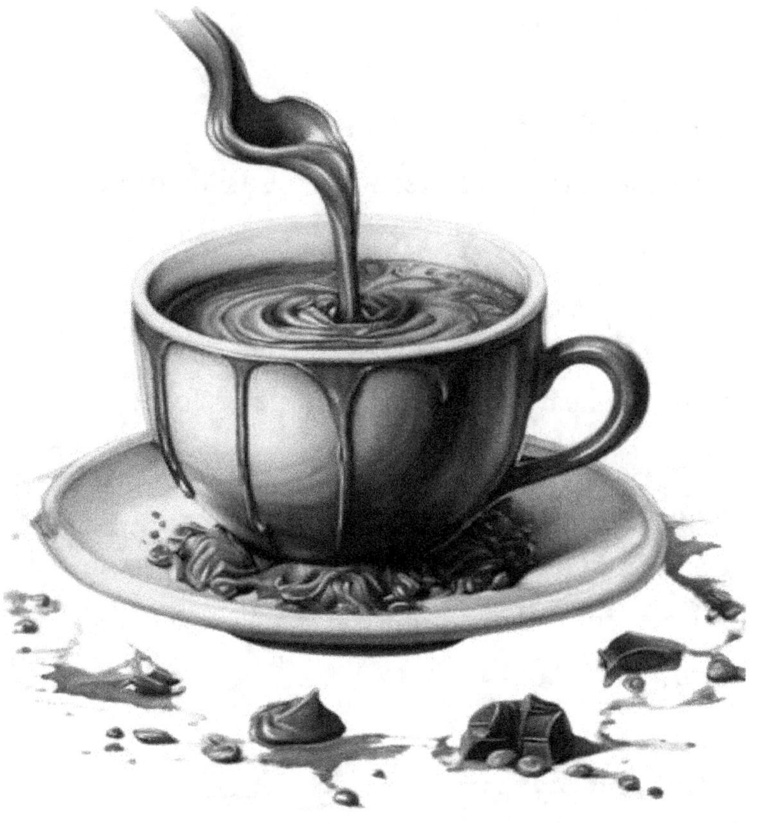

creating indulgent treats packed with potential health benefits. Adjust the quantity of mushroom extract to suit your taste preference and enjoy these unique chocolate creations!

Chapter 3: Crafting Mushroom Coffee Elixirs

3.1 Understanding the Coffee Bean: Selection and Preparation

Understanding coffee beans involves a nuanced exploration of their selection and preparation, fundamental to crafting the perfect cup of coffee. From sourcing to brewing, each step influences the richness, flavor, and aromatic profile of the final brew.

SOURCING QUALITY BEANS:

Selecting premium coffee beans sets the foundation for exceptional coffee. Consider factors like origin, variety, and roast level:

Origin:

Coffee beans from various regions exhibit unique flavors. For instance, Ethiopian beans might offer fruity and floral notes, while beans from Colombia might present a balanced acidity.

Variety:

Different coffee varieties—Arabica and Robusta—are distinct in taste and caffeine content. Arabica is celebrated for its nuanced flavors and lower caffeine, while Robusta tends to be more robust with higher caffeine content.

Roast Level:

Beans undergo various roast levels, from light to dark. Lighter roasts preserve bean flavors, while darker roasts offer richer, smokier profiles.

Grinding and Brewing:

Proper grinding and brewing methods are critical to extract the beans' flavors effectively:

Grind Consistency:

Grind beans to a consistent size suitable for the brewing method. Finer grinds suit espresso, while coarser grinds are ideal for French press or pour-over.

BREWING TECHNIQUE:

Match brewing techniques with coffee preferences. Experiment with methods like pour-over, French press, espresso machines, or cold brewing to accentuate specific flavor profiles.

STORAGE AND FRESHNESS:

Maintaining bean freshness ensures optimal flavor retention:

Storage: Store beans in airtight containers away from light, moisture, and heat to preserve freshness and prevent flavor degradation.

Freshness: Ideally, use beans within two weeks of roasting for peak freshness. Avoid pre-ground coffee as it loses flavor faster.

Understanding the nuances of coffee beans—from sourcing quality beans to precise grinding and brewing techniques—empowers enthusiasts to elevate their coffee experience. Appreciating the intricacies of bean selection and preparation leads to the creation of a flavorful, aromatic, and personalized cup of coffee, enriching every sip with a delightful coffee journey.

3.2 Methods of Infusing Mushrooms into Coffee Blends

Infusing mushrooms into coffee blends introduces a unique dimension to the beloved beverage, merging the rich flavors of coffee with

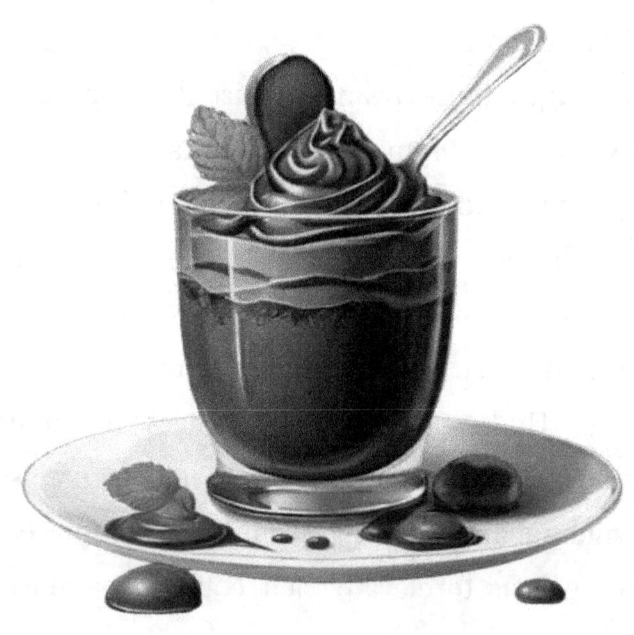

the potential health benefits of various mushroom varieties.

HERE'S A STEP-BY-STEP GUIDE ON INFUSING MUSHROOMS INTO COFFEE:

INGREDIENTS NEEDED:

Freshly ground coffee beans

Mushroom extract or powdered mushroom of choice (such as lion's mane, reishi, or chaga)

Optional:

Sweeteners, spices, or milk alternatives

STEP-BY-STEP INFUSION PROCESS:

Preparation of Mushroom Extract:

Start by preparing your preferred mushroom extract or powder according to the recommended instructions.

Ensure it is brewed or processed to extract its beneficial compounds.

Brewing Coffee:

Brew your coffee using your preferred method. This can be a drip coffee maker, French press, pour-over, or espresso machine.

Mushroom Infusion:

Once the coffee is brewed and ready, add the desired amount of mushroom extract or powder to the freshly brewed coffee. Start with a small quantity and adjust to taste.

Stirring and Mixing:

Stir the coffee thoroughly to ensure the mushroom extract or powder is well mixed and incorporated into the coffee.

Optional Additions:

If desired, add sweeteners like honey, spices like cinnamon, or milk alternatives to enhance the flavor profile further.

Enjoy Your Infused Coffee:

Pour the mushroom-infused coffee into your favorite mug and savor the unique blend of coffee flavors and potential health benefits from the mushrooms.

TIPS:

Experiment with different mushroom varieties and coffee ratios to achieve your preferred taste and potency.

Adjust the amount of mushroom extract or powder according to your desired level of mushroom flavor and potential health benefits. Store any leftover mushroom extract or powdered mushrooms in airtight containers for future use.

This method of infusing mushrooms into coffee offers an innovative way to elevate your coffee experience, combining the comforting aroma and taste of coffee with the potential wellness attributes of mushrooms.

HERE ARE RECIPES FOR MUSHROOM-ENHANCED COFFEES, LATTES, AND ENERGIZING ELIXIRS:

MUSHROOM-ENHANCED COFFEE:

INGREDIENTS:

1 cup freshly brewed coffee

1 teaspoon mushroom extract (choose from reishi, lion's mane, or chaga)

Optional:

Sweeteners (honey, maple syrup), spices (cinnamon, nutmeg), or milk alternatives

INSTRUCTIONS:

Brew Coffee:

Brew your favorite coffee using a preferred method—drip, French press, or espresso.

Add Mushroom Extract:

Pour the freshly brewed coffee into a mug and add the desired amount of mushroom extract. Stir well to combine.

Optional Additions:

Enhance the flavor by adding sweeteners like honey or maple syrup, spices such as cinnamon or nutmeg, or your preferred milk alternative.

Enjoy:

Sip and savor the rich flavors of the mushroom-enhanced coffee while potentially benefiting from the added wellness properties.

MUSHROOM LATTE:

INGREDIENTS:

1 cup steamed milk or milk alternative (oat, almond, coconut)

1 shot of espresso or 1 cup strong brewed coffee

1 teaspoon mushroom powder or extract (reishi, lion's mane)

Optional:

Sweeteners (agave, maple syrup), spices (cocoa, turmeric), or whipped cream for topping

INSTRUCTIONS:

Brew Espresso or Coffee:

Prepare a shot of espresso or brew strong coffee.

Prepare Milk:

Steam your preferred milk or milk alternative until frothy.

Mix Ingredients:

In a mug, combine the brewed espresso or coffee with the mushroom extract or powder. Stir well.

Pour Steamed Milk:

Gently pour the steamed frothy milk over the mushroom-coffee mixture.

Optional Additions and Serve:

Add sweeteners or spices as desired. Top with whipped cream or a sprinkle of cocoa for an extra touch.

ENERGIZING MUSHROOM ELIXIR:

INGREDIENTS:

1 cup brewed adaptogenic tea (like ginseng or holy basil)

1 teaspoon mushroom powder (cordyceps, chaga)

1 tablespoon honey or agave syrup

Dash of cinnamon or ginger (optional)

INSTRUCTIONS:

Brew Adaptogenic Tea:

Brew a cup of adaptogenic tea, such as ginseng or holy basil, according to package instructions.

Mix Ingredients:

In a mug, combine the brewed tea with the mushroom powder. Stir until well incorporated.

Add Sweetener and Spice:

Add honey or agave syrup for sweetness. Optionally, sprinkle a dash of cinnamon or ginger for flavor.

Enjoy:

Sip slowly and revel in the potential energizing effects of this mushroom-enhanced elixir.

These recipes offer delightful ways to incorporate mushroom extracts or powders into your daily coffee routine, adding unique flavors and potential wellness benefits to your favorite beverages. Adjust ingredients to suit your taste preferences and enjoy the aromatic journey!

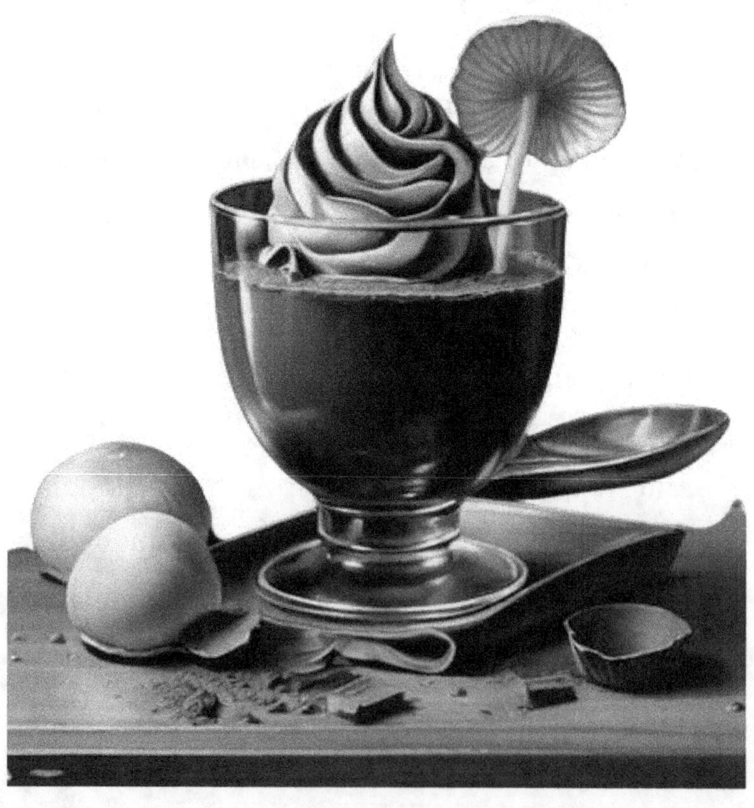

Chapter 4: The Science Behind Mushroom Benefits

4.1 Exploring the Nutritional and Medicinal Value of Mushrooms

Exploring the nutritional and medicinal value of mushrooms unveils a treasure trove of benefits, showcasing these fungi as more than just culinary delights. Various mushroom species offer unique nutritional profiles and medicinal properties, contributing to overall well-being:

NUTRITIONAL VALUE:

MACRONUTRIENTS:

Protein: Mushrooms contain varying amounts of protein, providing essential amino acids necessary for bodily functions.

Carbohydrates: They offer carbohydrates like chitin and beta-glucans, aiding in digestion and potentially supporting the immune system.

Fiber: Rich in dietary fiber, mushrooms contribute to digestive health and may help regulate cholesterol levels.

MICRONUTRIENTS:

Vitamins: Abundant in vitamins like B-complex (riboflavin, niacin, pantothenic acid), supporting energy production and nerve function. Some varieties also contain vitamin D.

Minerals: Potassium, selenium, copper, and phosphorus are among the minerals found in mushrooms, supporting various bodily processes.

How Mushroom Compounds Enhance Health and Wellness

Mushroom compounds exhibit a fascinating array of properties that contribute to enhancing health and wellness. These compounds, found in various mushroom species, offer a spectrumof benefits that positively impact different aspects of well-being:

BETA-GLUCANS:

Immune Support: Beta-glucans, abundant in mushrooms like reishi and shiitake, possess immune-modulating properties. They stimulate immune cells, potentially enhancing the body's defense against infections and diseases.

POLYSACCHARIDES:

Antioxidant Activity: Polysaccharides found in mushrooms act as antioxidants, combating oxidative stress and free radicals. This activity may reduce inflammation and cellular damage, contributing to overall health.

TRITERPENES AND TRITERPENOIDS:

Anti-Inflammatory Effects: Compounds like triterpenes in mushrooms such as chaga and reishi exhibit anti-inflammatory properties, potentially alleviating inflammation-related conditions.

ERGOTHIONEINE:

Cellular Protection: Ergothioneine, present in some mushroom varieties like oyster mushrooms, acts as a potent antioxidant, protecting cells from damage caused by oxidative stress.

ADAPTOGENS:

Stress Management: Certain mushrooms like cordyceps and lion's mane possess adaptogenic properties. These compounds potentially aid the body in managing stress, supporting resilience, and balancing physiological responses.

NEUROTROPHIC FACTORS:

Brain Health: Compounds in lion's mane mushrooms may stimulate the production of nerve growth factor (NGF), crucial for nerve cell maintenance and potentially aiding cognitive function.

INCORPORATING MUSHROOM COMPOUNDS:

Dietary Inclusions: Including a variety of mushrooms in the diet or consuming mushroom extracts and supplements provides access to these beneficial compounds.

Holistic Practices: Integrating mushrooms into holistic health practices, such as traditional medicine or supplements, may leverage their potential wellness benefits.

Understanding how mushroom compounds enhance health and wellness highlights their diverse contributions.

From immune support and antioxidant properties to stress management and cognitive health, these compounds offer a multifaceted approach to fostering overall well-being, making mushrooms an intriguing component of holistic health and nutrition.

4.2 Dosage Recommendations and Safety Considerations

DOSAGE RECOMMENDATIONS:

1. Consider Product Specifics:

Dosage guidelines can vary depending on the type of mushroom supplement or extract being used. Follow manufacturer recommendations for dosage and usage.

2. Start Conservatively:

Begin with a lower dosage and gradually increase as needed. Monitor how your body responds to the supplement.

3. Consult a Healthcare Professional:

Seek advice from a healthcare provider or a qualified herbalist/naturopathic doctor for personalized dosage recommendations, especially if you have underlying health conditions or are taking other medications.

4. Follow Established Guidelines:

In the absence of specific recommendations, general guidelines suggest a range of doses. For instance, a typical dose might range from 500mg to 2000mg per day, but this can vary based on the mushroom type and extract concentration.

SAFETY CONSIDERATIONS:

1. Allergies and Sensitivities:

Individuals with known allergies to mushrooms or specific types of fungi should avoid mushroom supplements to prevent adverse reactions.

2. Quality and Purity:

Ensure the supplement is sourced from reputable brands with quality control measures to ensure purity and safety. Look for third-party certifications if available.

3. Potential Interactions:

Some mushroom supplements may interact with certain medications. Consult a healthcare professional before starting mushroom supplementation if you're on medications.

4. Adverse Effects:

While rare, some individuals might experience mild side effects such as digestive issues or allergic reactions. Discontinue use and consult a healthcare professional if adverse effects occur.

5. Pregnancy and Breastfeeding:
Pregnant or breastfeeding individuals should avoid mushroom supplements unless advised otherwise by a healthcare provider due to limited safety data in these populations.

Mushroom supplements and extracts can be valuable additions to a wellness routine when used judiciously and with proper consideration for individual health factors. Adhering to recommended dosages, seeking professional guidance, and being mindful of safety precautions can help optimize the benefits while minimizing potential risks. Always prioritize safety and informed decision-making when incorporating any supplements into your health regimen.

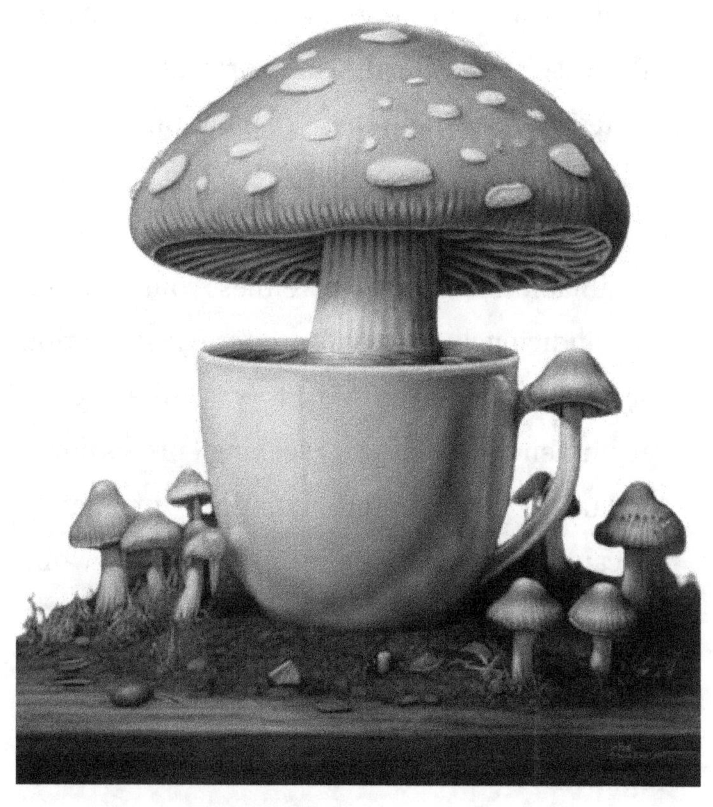

Chapter 5: Culinary Innovation with Mushrooms

5.1 Beyond Chocolate and Coffee: Mushroom-Infused Snacks and Beverages

Exploring the realm of mushroom-infused snacks and beverages unveils a diverse array of innovative culinary creations that extend beyond traditional uses in chocolate and coffee. Incorporating mushrooms into various snacks and beverages offers unique flavors, nutritional benefits, and potential wellness enhancements:

MUSHROOM-INFUSED SNACKS:

1. Trail Mixes:

Blend dried mushrooms like shiitake or porcini into trail mixes for a savory twist. Combine with nuts, seeds, and dried fruits for a wholesome and flavorful snack.

2. Popcorn Seasoning:

Create savory popcorn by sprinkling powdered mushroom extracts (such as reishi or lion's mane) mixed with herbs and spices for an umami-packed snack.

3. Mushroom Chips:

Thinly slice mushrooms like oyster or portobello, season them, and bake or dehydrate to create crispy and nutritious mushroom chips.

4. Energy Balls or Bars:

Incorporate powdered mushroom extracts into homemade energy balls or bars for a boost of nutrients and potential adaptogenic benefits.

MUSHROOM-INFUSED BEVERAGES:

1. Tea Blends:

Blend mushroom extracts or dried mushrooms with herbal teas to create unique, earthy-infused tea blends. Pair with complementary herbs for enhanced flavor.

2. Smoothies or Juices:

Add mushroom extracts or powdered mushrooms to smoothies or fresh juices for an additional nutrient boost without compromising taste.

3. Mushroom Mocktails:

Experiment with mushroom extracts to craft non-alcoholic beverages or mocktails, infusing unique flavors into refreshing drinks.

4. Sparkling Mushroom Waters:

Combine mushroom extracts with sparkling water and natural sweeteners for effervescent and hydrating mushroom-infused beverages.

BENEFITS OF DIVERSIFYING MUSHROOM INFUSIONS:

Flavor Innovation: Expanding mushroom infusions into snacks and beverages offers diverse tastes, catering to savory and sweet preferences.

Nutritional Boost: These creations provide an alternative way to incorporate the potential health benefits of mushrooms into daily snacks or hydration routines.

Culinary Versatility: Mushroom-infused snacks and beverages open avenues for culinary experimentation, offering new ways to enjoy the rich flavors and potential wellness properties of mushrooms.

The extension of mushroom infusions beyond traditional realms like chocolate and coffee into a broader spectrum of snacks and beverages showcases the versatility of mushrooms in enhancing flavors, nutritional profiles, and potential wellness benefits. Embracing these innovative creations invites a world of culinary exploration while potentially harnessing the health-enhancing properties of mushrooms in everyday indulgences.

HOMEMADE MUSHROOM COFFEE:

Mushroom Extract Dosage:
Start with 0.5 to 1 teaspoon: This is a common starting point for incorporating mushroom extract or powdered mushrooms into your coffee.

Gradually Increase: Depending on the desired strength and flavor, gradually increase the amount of mushroom extract or powder.

COFFEE DOSAGE:
Regular Coffee Ratio: Use your preferred amount of brewed coffee, maintaining the standard coffee-to-water ratio based on your taste preferences.

Adjust to Taste: Add the mushroom extract or powder to the brewed coffee and adjust according to taste preferences. Some may prefer a subtle hint of mushroom flavor, while others may prefer a more pronounced taste.

HOMEMADE MUSHROOM CHOCOLATE:

Mushroom Powder Dosage:

0.5 to 1 teaspoon per serving: When incorporating mushroom powder into homemade chocolate, start with a conservative amount.

Experiment Gradually: Adjust the quantity of mushroom powder based on desired taste and potential health benefits.

Chocolate Base:

Adapt Based on Recipe: Follow the recipe for making chocolate bars, truffles, or any chocolate-based treats, incorporating the mushroom powder or extract.

Balance Flavor and Health: Incorporate enough mushroom powder to derive potential benefits while ensuring the chocolate maintains its desired flavor profile.

SAFETY AND CONSULTATION:

Consultation: For personalized dosage recommendations and potential interactions, especially if you have existing health conditions or are on medications, consult with a healthcare professional or a qualified herbalist/naturopathic doctor.

Start Conservatively: Begin with lower amounts and gradually increase to ensure tolerance and assess any potential effects on taste and health.

While these dosage suggestions offer a starting point, individual tolerance, preferences, and the specific mushroom used can influence the ideal dosage. Adjustments should be made based on personal preferences and health considerations, and seeking professional advice is advisable for personalized recommendations.

5.2   Savory   Mushroom-Infused Dishes and Entrees

Exploring savory mushroom-infused dishes and entrees introduces a world of culinary creativity, enhancing flavors and nutritional profiles. Incorporating mushrooms into savory recipes adds depth, umami richness, and potential health benefits to a diverse range of meals:

MUSHROOM-INFUSED DISHES:

1. Mushroom Risotto:
Technique: Use a variety of mushrooms like porcini, shiitake, or cremini to enrich the creamy texture and earthy flavors of the risotto. Incorporate mushroom broth or mushroom extract for an added depth of taste.

2. Stuffed Mushrooms:

Preparation: Hollow out mushroom caps and fill them with a savory mixture of breadcrumbs, cheese, herbs, and chopped mushroom stems. Bake until golden for a flavorful appetizer.

3. Mushroom Gravy or Sauce:

Complement: Prepare a robust mushroom-based gravy or sauce using a blend of mushrooms, onions, garlic, and broth. Serve it over roasted vegetables, meats, or mashed potatoes for a rich accompaniment.

4. Mushroom Tacos or Burritos:

Filling Enhancement: Sauté sliced mushrooms with onions, peppers, and taco seasoning for a vegetarian-friendly, umami-filled taco or burrito filling.

MUSHROOM-INFUSED ENTREES:

1. Mushroom Wellington:

Elegant Dish: Use a mix of finely chopped mushrooms, herbs, and shallots wrapped in puff pastry for a sophisticated vegetarian main course.

2. Mushroom Pasta Dishes:

Flavorful Additions: Incorporate mushrooms into pasta dishes like creamy mushroom fettuccine or mushroom and garlic spaghetti for a hearty and satisfying meal.

3. Mushroom Stir-Fry:

Quick and Versatile: Stir-fry sliced mushrooms with assorted vegetables, tofu, or meat in a flavorful sauce for a nutrient-packed and quick dinner option.

4. Mushroom-Based Soups:

Hearty and Warming: Prepare mushroom-based soups like creamy mushroom bisque or wild mushroom soup for a comforting and flavorsome starter or main dish.

BENEFITS OF SAVORY MUSHROOM DISHES:

Rich Umami Flavor: Mushrooms offer a natural umami taste, enhancing the overall depth and richness of savory dishes.

Nutritional Boost: Incorporating mushrooms introduces additional nutrients, such as B-vitamins, minerals, and potential health-promoting compounds, into meals.

Vegetarian and Versatile: Mushrooms can serve as a substantial and satisfying substitute for meat in vegetarian or vegan dishes, offering a variety of cooking possibilities.

Savory mushroom-infused dishes and entrees showcase the versatility and culinary potential of mushrooms in creating delicious and nutritionally rich meals. Whether as a complementing ingredient or the star of the dish, mushrooms add depth and complexity to savory culinary creations while potentially contributing to a wholesome and flavorful dining experience.

FUSION RECIPES BLENDING MUSHROOMS WITH OTHER INGREDIENTS

Fusion recipes that combine mushrooms with other ingredients offer an exciting culinary adventure, merging flavors and textures to create innovative and delicious dishes.

HERE ARE CREATIVE FUSION RECIPES INCORPORATING MUSHROOMS:

MUSHROOM-PESTO PIZZA:

Ingredients:

Pizza dough

Pesto sauce

Sliced mushrooms (shiitake, cremini)

Mozzarella cheese

Fresh basil leaves

Instructions:

Prepare Pizza Base: Roll out the pizza dough and spread a layer of pesto sauce as the base.

Add Mushrooms: Arrange sliced mushrooms evenly over the pesto sauce.

Top with Cheese: Sprinkle mozzarella cheese generously over the mushrooms.

Bake: Bake in a preheated oven until the crust is golden and the cheese is bubbly.

Garnish: Finish with fresh basil leaves for added freshness and aroma.

MUSHROOM-SPINACH QUESADILLAS:

Ingredients:

Flour tortillas

Sautéed mushrooms (portobello, oyster)

Fresh spinach leaves

Shredded cheese (cheddar, Monterey Jack)

Olive oil

Instructions:

Assemble Quesadillas: Layer sautéed mushrooms, fresh spinach leaves, and shredded cheese on a tortilla.

Fold and Cook: Fold the tortilla in half and cook in a lightly oiled pan until golden brown on both sides.

Slice and Serve: Cut the quesadilla into wedges and serve with salsa or guacamole.

MUSHROOM-CAULIFLOWER CURRY:

Ingredients:

Chopped mushrooms (button, porcini)

Cauliflower florets

Curry paste or powder

Coconut milk

Onion, garlic, ginger

Fresh cilantro for garnish

Instructions:

Sauté Aromatics: Sauté onion, garlic, and ginger in a pan until fragrant.

Add Mushrooms and Cauliflower: Add chopped mushrooms and cauliflower florets to the pan and cook until slightly tender.

Season and Simmer: Stir in curry paste or powder, pour in coconut milk, and simmer until vegetables are cooked through and the flavors meld.

Serve: Garnish with fresh cilantro and serve with rice or naan.

BENEFITS OF FUSION RECIPES:

Creativity and Innovation: Fusion cooking offers a platform for experimenting with diverse ingredients, resulting in unique and flavorful combinations.

Cultural Diversity: Blending ingredients from different culinary traditions allows for cultural exchange and diverse taste experiences.

Nutritional Diversity: Combining mushrooms with various ingredients brings together different nutrients and flavors in a single dish.

Fusion recipes that blend mushrooms with other ingredients showcase the versatility of mushrooms and their ability to harmonize with various flavors and cuisines. These innovative combinations not only offer delicious meals but also present opportunities to explore new culinary dimensions, embracing diversity and creativity in the kitchen.

Chapter 6: Wellness and Mushroom Consumption

6.1 Understanding Mushroom-Driven Wellness: Mental and Physical Health Benefits

Understanding the comprehensive wellness contributions of mushrooms reveals their potential to positively impact both mental and physical health, offering an array of benefits:

MENTAL HEALTH BENEFITS:

1. Cognitive Support:

Certain mushrooms, like lion's mane, are believed to support cognitive function by potentially enhancing nerve growth factor (NGF) production. This may aid memory and concentration.

2. Stress Management:

Adaptogenic mushrooms, including reishi and cordyceps, have properties that may help the body adapt to stressors, potentially promoting resilience and reducing the impact of stress.

3. Mood Regulation:

Compounds found in mushrooms, such as beta-glucans, may have a positive impact on mood regulation by potentially modulating immune responses that affect mood.

PHYSICAL HEALTH BENEFITS:

1. Immune Support:

Beta-glucans and other compounds in mushrooms, particularly varieties like shiitake and maitake, may enhance immune function, aiding in defense against infections.

2. Anti-Inflammatory Effects:

Certain mushrooms, like chaga and reishi, contain compounds that exhibit anti-inflammatory properties, potentially reducing inflammation and supporting overall health.

3. Antioxidant Properties:

Mushrooms are rich in antioxidants like ergothioneine and polyphenols, which combat oxidative stress, potentially reducing cell damage and supporting cellular health.

HOLISTIC WELLNESS:

1. Gut Health:

Mushrooms contain prebiotic fibers that may support gut health by promoting beneficial gut bacteria, contributing to overall digestive wellness.

2. Nutritional Density:

Mushrooms offer a spectrum of nutrients, including vitamins (B-complex, vitamin D), minerals (selenium, potassium), and protein, contributing to a balanced diet and overall wellness.

Mushrooms' wellness benefits encompass both mental and physical health realms, showcasing their potential as a holistic addition to wellness routines. From cognitive support and stress management to immune enhancement and anti-inflammatory properties, mushrooms offer a diverse range of contributions. Embracing mushrooms as a part of a balanced diet and holistic wellness approach can potentially promote overall well-being, both mentally and physically.

6.2 Incorporating Mushrooms for Stress Relief, Immunity, and Overall Well-Being

Incorporating mushrooms into your daily routine can significantly contribute to stress relief, bolstered immunity, and overall well-being, thanks to their diverse range of health-supporting compounds:

STRESS RELIEF:

1. Adaptogenic Properties:
Certain mushrooms like reishi, cordyceps, and lion's mane possess adaptogenic properties, potentially aiding the body in adapting to stressors and supporting stress management.

2. Calmative Effects:
Compounds found in mushrooms, such as beta-glucans and polysaccharides, may exert calming effects, helping to alleviate stress and promote relaxation.

IMMUNE SUPPORT:

1. Enhanced Immune Function:
Mushrooms like shiitake, maitake, and reishi are rich in beta-glucans, known for their immune-modulating properties that can potentially enhance the body's defense against infections.

2. Antioxidant Defense:

The antioxidant compounds in mushrooms, such as ergothioneine and polyphenols, contribute to reducing oxidative stress, fortifying the immune system against cellular damage.

OVERALL WELL-BEING:

1. Nutrient-Rich Profile:

Mushrooms offer a spectrum of nutrients, including vitamins (B-complex, vitamin D), minerals (selenium, potassium), and proteins, supporting overall health and vitality.

2. Gut Health Support:

Mushrooms contain prebiotic fibers that nourish beneficial gut bacteria, promoting a healthy gut microbiome, which is crucial for overall well-being.

PRACTICAL INCORPORATION:

1. Dietary Inclusions:

Integrate various mushroom varieties into meals—whether in soups, stir-fries, or as standalone dishes—to benefit from their diverse nutrients and potential health properties.

2. Supplements or Extracts:

Consider incorporating mushroom extracts or supplements into your routine, ensuring they are sourced from reputable brands to benefit from concentrated mushroom compounds.

Incorporating mushrooms into your diet or supplement routine can serve as a valuable strategy for stress relief, immunity enhancement, and overall well-being. These versatile fungi offer a range of health-supporting compounds that contribute to a holistic approach to health, providing numerous opportunities to leverage their potential benefits for an enhanced sense of wellness.

6.3 Balancing Dosage and Incorporating Mushrooms into Daily Regimens

Achieving a balanced and effective dosage when incorporating mushrooms into daily regimens is crucial to optimize their potential benefits while ensuring safety and well-being:

UNDERSTANDING DOSAGE:

1. Start Conservatively:
Begin with a lower dosage to assess individual tolerance and response to mushroom supplements or extracts. Gradually increase as needed.

2. Follow Recommended Guidelines:
Adhere to manufacturer's recommendations or dosage guidelines provided by qualified healthcare professionals for specific mushroom types and products.

3. Consider Individual Factors:

Personal health status, age, weight, and existing medications can influence the ideal dosage. Seek professional advice for tailored recommendations.

METHODS OF INCORPORATION:

1. Dietary Integration:

Introduce a variety of mushrooms into meals regularly. Cooked or raw, mushrooms can be added to soups, stir-fries, salads, and other dishes for diverse nutritional intake.

2. Supplements or Extracts:

Utilize mushroom extracts or supplements from reputable sources. Follow the suggested dosage and frequency outlined on the product packaging or as advised by a healthcare professional.

3. Monitor Effects:

Pay attention to how your body responds to the dosage. Observe any changes in mood, energy levels, digestion, or overall well-being to adjust dosage if needed.

ENSURING SAFETY:

1. Consultation with Professionals:

Seek guidance from healthcare providers, herbalists, or nutritionists for personalized recommendations, especially if managing specific health conditions or on medications.

2. Quality Assurance:

Choose high-quality mushroom supplements or extracts from reputable brands, ensuring purity, potency, and absence of contaminants.

3. Adherence to Guidelines:

Adhere strictly to recommended dosages and avoid exceeding the suggested amounts to prevent potential adverse effects or interactions.

Balancing dosage and integrating mushrooms into daily regimens involves understanding individual needs, following recommended guidelines, and prioritizing safety. Whether through dietary incorporation or supplements, maintaining a balanced approach and seeking professional advice can optimize the benefits of mushrooms while promoting overall well-being. Regular assessment and adjustments to dosage can help ensure a harmonious integration of mushrooms into daily health routines.

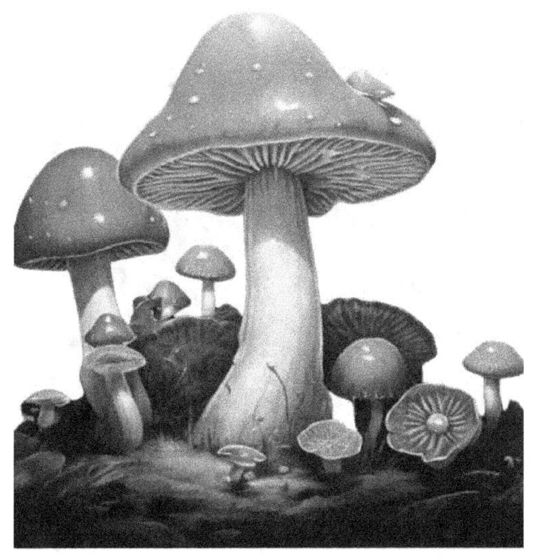

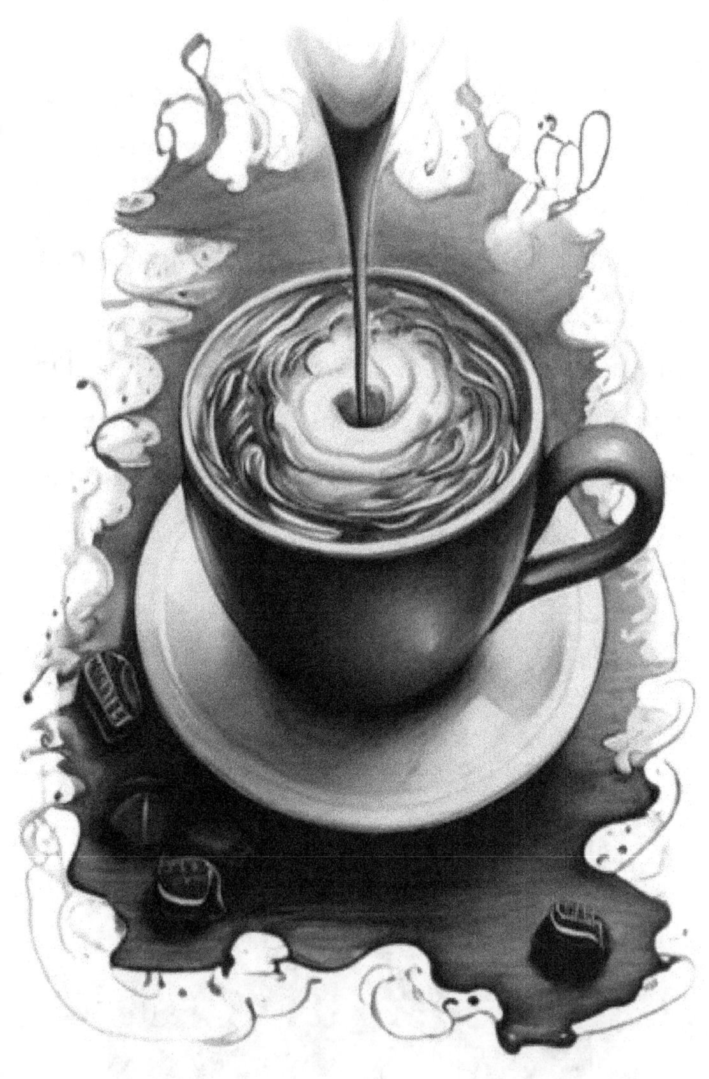

Chapter 7: Crafting Your Elixirs at Home

7.1 Step-by-Step Guide to Crafting Mushroom Chocolate and Coffee Infusions

MUSHROOM CHOCOLATE INFUSION:

Ingredients:

Dark chocolate (bars or chips)

Mushroom powder or extract (e.g., reishi, lion's mane)

Double boiler or microwave-safe bowl

Silicone molds or parchment-lined tray

Steps:

Prepare Chocolate:

Break the dark chocolate into smaller pieces and place them in a clean, dry double boiler or microwave-safe bowl.

Melt Chocolate:

Use the double boiler method or microwave the bowl in short bursts, stirring occasionally until the chocolate melts smoothly.

Incorporate Mushroom Extract:

Once the chocolate is melted, add the desired amount of mushroom powder or extract. Start with a small amount and gradually increase based on taste preference and desired potency.

Mix Thoroughly:

Stir the mushroom extract into the melted chocolate until it is evenly combined. Ensure there are no lumps and the infusion is well distributed.

Pour into Molds:

Pour the mushroom-infused chocolate mixture into silicone molds or onto a parchment-lined tray, spreading it evenly with a spatula.

Set and Solidify:

Allow the chocolate to set and solidify at room temperature or place it in the refrigerator for quicker solidification.

Unmold and Store:

Once solidified, carefully remove the mushroom-infused chocolate from the molds. Store it in an airtight container in a cool, dry place.

MUSHROOM COFFEE INFUSION:

Ingredients:

Coffee beans (whole or ground)

Mushroom coffee powder or extract (e.g., chaga, cordyceps)

Coffee grinder (if using whole beans)

Filtered water

French press, coffee maker, or preferred brewing equipment

Steps:

Prepare Coffee:

Grind the coffee beans to your preferred consistency if using whole beans.

Brew Coffee:

Brew your regular coffee using a French press, coffee maker, or preferred brewing method.

Add Mushroom Infusion:

Once the coffee is brewed, add the recommended amount of mushroom coffee powder or extract to the brewed coffee. Start with a small amount and adjust based on taste preference.

Stir Well:

Stir the mushroom coffee infusion thoroughly to ensure the mushroom powder or extract blends completely with the coffee.

Enjoy:

Pour the mushroom-infused coffee into your favorite mug and savor the unique flavors and potential health benefits.

Crafting mushroom-infused chocolate and coffee involves combining quality ingredients with mushroom extracts or powders, ensuring thorough mixing, and enjoying the unique flavors and potential wellness enhancements they offer. Adjust the amounts of mushroom extracts based on personal taste preferences and desired potency.

7.2 Tips for Sourcing Quality Ingredients and Mushrooms

When sourcing ingredients and mushrooms for culinary or wellness purposes, here are some tips to ensure you obtain high-quality products:

TIPS FOR SOURCING QUALITY INGREDIENTS:

1. Choose Organic when Possible:

Opt for organic ingredients, such as dark chocolate or coffee beans, to minimize exposure to pesticides and ensure higher quality.

2. Check Labels and Certifications:

Look for certifications like USDA Organic, Fair Trade, or other reputable certifications that guarantee quality and ethical sourcing practices.

3. Consider Sustainable and Ethical Practices:

Support brands or suppliers that prioritize sustainability, fair trade practices, and ethical sourcing of ingredients.

4. Freshness and Storage:

Ensure the ingredients, especially coffee beans and chocolate, are fresh and properly stored in airtight containers away from moisture, heat, and light.

TIPS FOR SOURCING QUALITY MUSHROOMS:

1. Choose Reputable Suppliers:

Purchase mushrooms from trusted and reputable suppliers, whether local farmers' markets, certified organic stores, or reputable online sources.

2. Quality of Mushrooms:

Look for mushrooms that are fresh, firm, and free from signs of spoilage, molds, or discoloration. Dried mushrooms should be intact and fragrant.

3. Consider Mushroom Varieties:

Select specific mushroom varieties known for their medicinal or culinary benefits, such as reishi, lion's mane, chaga, or cordyceps, from reliable sources.

4. Certified and Lab-Tested Products:

Choose mushroom products that are certified, lab-tested for purity, and free from contaminants to ensure safety and quality.

ADDITIONAL CONSIDERATIONS:

1. Research and Reviews:
Conduct research and read reviews about the brands or suppliers to gauge the quality and reliability of their products.

2. Ethical Harvesting Practices:
Choose suppliers who engage in ethical harvesting practices and sustainable cultivation methods for mushrooms.

3. Consult Experts:
When unsure, consult with experts, nutritionists, or herbalists for recommendations on trusted sources and quality mushroom products.

Sourcing quality ingredients and mushrooms involves considering factors like organic certification, freshness, ethical practices, and reputable suppliers. By prioritizing reputable brands, certifications, and freshness, consumers can ensure they're obtaining high-quality ingredients and mushrooms for culinary and wellness purposes.

Always prioritize safety, quality, and ethical sourcing when selecting ingredients and mushroom products.

7.3 Equipment, Techniques, and Storage Suggestions

Here's a comprehensive guide covering equipment, techniques, and storage suggestions for mushroom-infused products:

EQUIPMENT:

1. Double Boiler or Microwave-Safe Bowl:

Use a double boiler or a microwave-safe bowl for melting chocolate when making mushroom-infused chocolate.

2. Silicone Molds or Parchment-Lined Tray:

Use silicone molds or a parchment-lined tray for molding and shaping mushroom-infused chocolate into bars or shapes.

3. Coffee Grinder (if using whole beans):

If utilizing whole coffee beans for mushroom-infused coffee, a grinder ensures consistent grind size for brewing.

4. Brewing Equipment:

Employ a French press, coffee maker, or preferred brewing equipment for making mushroom-infused coffee.

TECHNIQUES:

1. Melting Chocolate:

Melt chocolate using a double boiler or microwave in short bursts, stirring occasionally until smooth.

2. Incorporating Mushroom Extracts:

Stir mushroom extracts or powders thoroughly into melted chocolate or brewed coffee until evenly blended.

3. Brewing Coffee:

Brew coffee as per usual, then add the recommended amount of mushroom coffee powder or extract.

4. Portion Control:

Start with smaller amounts of mushroom extracts and gradually increase to suit taste preferences and desired potency.

STORAGE SUGGESTIONS:

1. Mushroom-Infused Chocolate:

Store in an airtight container in a cool, dry place away from direct sunlight to prevent melting or spoilage.

2. Mushroom Coffee Infusion:

Store mushroom-infused coffee in a sealed container or resealable bag, away from moisture and heat to maintain freshness.

3. Mushroom Powders or Extracts:

Keep mushroom powders or extracts in airtight containers in a cool, dry place following the manufacturer's recommendations for storage.

4. Coffee Beans and Chocolate:

Store coffee beans in an airtight container away from heat and light. Store chocolate similarly, avoiding moisture and extreme temperatures.

ADDITIONAL TIPS:

1. Labeling and Dating:

Label containers with contents and dates to monitor freshness and potency.

2. Shelf Life Consideration:

Be mindful of shelf life; use mushroom-infused products within recommended timeframes for optimal quality.

3. Avoid Contamination:

Prevent cross-contamination by ensuring equipment and storage containers are clean and dry before use.

Utilizing appropriate equipment, techniques, and storage practices is crucial when crafting mushroom-infused products like chocolate and coffee. Proper storage in sealed containers, labeling, and using designated equipment ensures freshness and maintains the quality of the infused ingredients for longer durations. By employing these techniques and storage suggestions, enthusiasts can enjoy mushroom-infused delights at their best.

Conclusion

Encouraging Readers to Embrace Mushroom-Infused Culinary Adventures

Dear Culinary Enthusiasts,

Step into a world where culinary creativity meets the enchanting allure of mushrooms! Are you ready to embark on a flavorful journey that transcends ordinary dining experiences? The magic of mushrooms awaits, promising a symphony of tastes and a feast for the senses.

The Dance of Flavors:

Picture the velvety richness of dark chocolate entwined with the earthy undertones of mushrooms, or the invigorating aroma of freshly brewed coffee infused with the subtle notes of your favorite fungi. These are not just meals; they are culinary adventures waiting to be savored.

Wellness on Your Plate:

But it's not just about taste; it's about nourishing your body and soul. Discover the wellness secrets these remarkable fungi hold, offering immune support, stress relief, and a holistic approach to well-being. It's a culinary journey that transcends the ordinary and embraces the extraordinary.

Your Kitchen, Your Canvas:

In the heart of your kitchen, you hold the brush to paint a masterpiece of flavors. Experiment with mushroom-infused recipes, letting your taste buds be your guide. From delectable desserts to comforting beverages, the possibilities are as endless as your imagination.

Join the Culinary Revolution:

It's time to join the culinary revolution, where every meal is an opportunity for discovery. Embrace the versatility of mushrooms as they elevate your dishes to new heights, promising a harmonious blend of taste and nutrition

Dear reader,

As you savor the known, embrace the unknown. Let each meal be an opportunity to push boundaries, experiment fearlessly, and revel in the joy of culinary discovery.

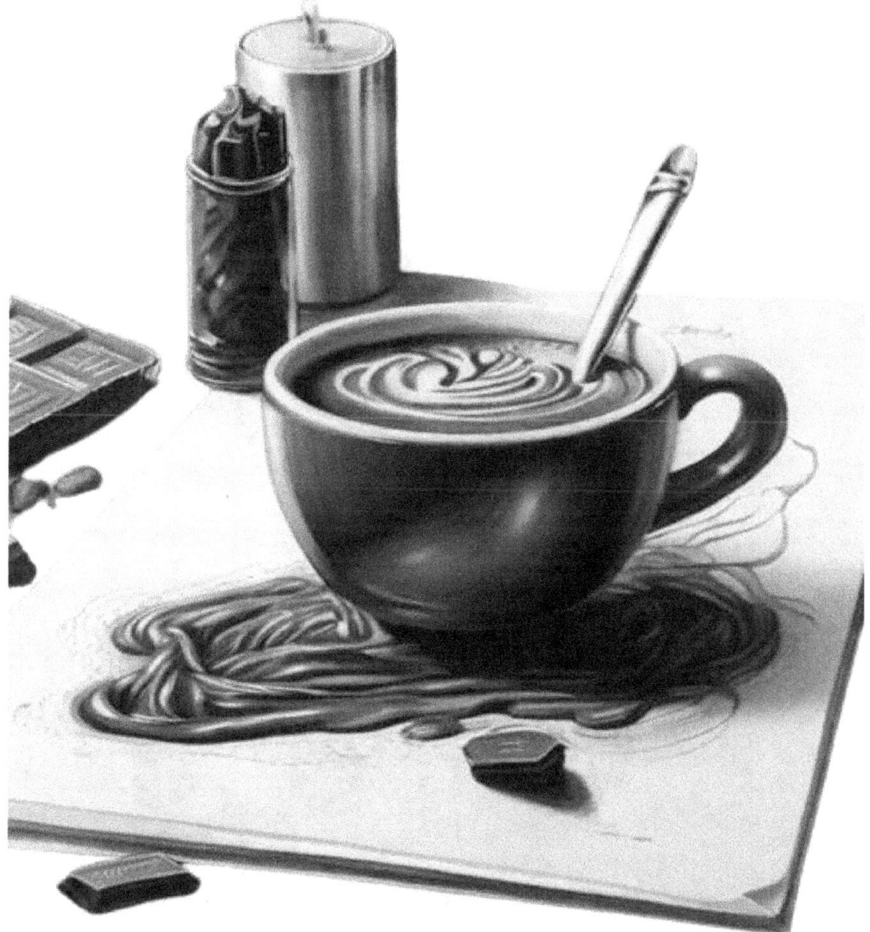

The world of mushrooms beckons, and your culinary journey has only just begun.

Here's to endless experimentation and a tapestry of flavors yet to be woven!

Happy exploring!
[A J BLAZE]

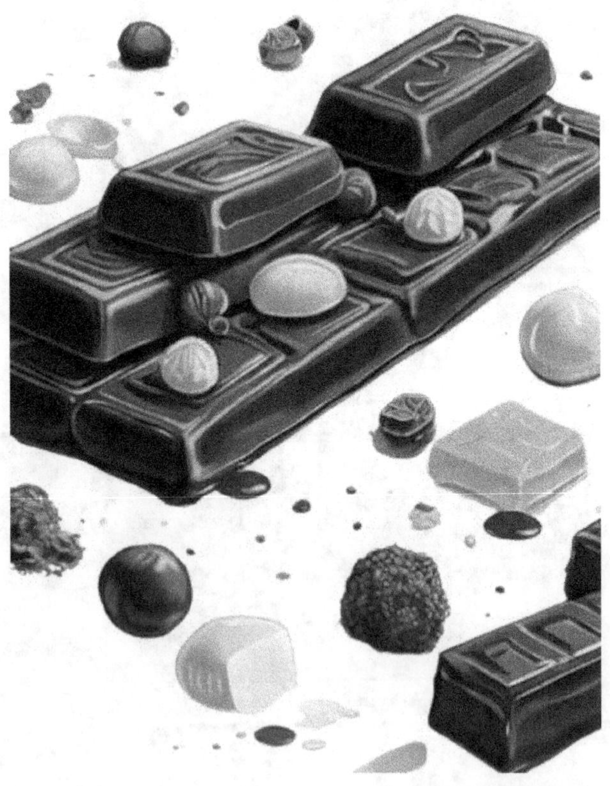

www.ingramcontent.com/pod-product-compliance
Lightning Source LLC
Chambersburg PA
CBHW050925260726
48660CB00001B/404